The Secret
Benefits of
lemon and
honey

The Secret
Benefits of
lemon and
honey

VIJAYA KUMAR

NEW DAWN PRESS, INC.
UK • USA • INDIA

NEW DAWN PRESS GROUP
Published by New Dawn Press Group
New Dawn Press, Inc., 244 South Randall Rd # 90, Elgin, IL 60123
e-mail: sales@newdawnpress.com

New Dawn Press, 2 Tintern Close, Slough, Berkshire, SL1-2TB, UK
e-mail: salesuk@newdawnpress.org

New Dawn Press (An Imprint of Sterling Publishers (P) Ltd)
A-59, Okhla Industrial Area, Phase-II, New Delhi-110020, India
E-mail: sterlingpublishers@airtelbroadband.in
www.sterlingpublishers.com

The Secret Benefits of lemon and honey
© 2007, Sterling Publishers (P) Ltd
ISBN 978-1-84557-838-1

PRINTED IN INDIA

Contents

Introduction

Using the simplest of ingredients, lemon and honey, this book offers alternative methods of treatment and prevention of a wide range of diseases and nagging complaints that often deny conventional diagnosis and treatment.

Traditionally used in our kitchen, today lemon and honey are found as ingredients in various cosmetics, fragrant baths, healing teas, refreshing drinks, and vitamin-rich juices. They are also commonly used in health care clinics. Each part of the lemon – pulp, peel and essential oil – are useful. Honey as well as the waxy comb from the honey comb have rejuvenating properties. The combined effect of lemon and honey brings vigour and vitality to your daily being.

Essence of Lemon and Honey

Lemon

In ancient days Egyptians used lemon for its healing properties and also as an aphrodisiac.

In the Middle-East and South-West Asia there was a general belief that eating lemon and drinking its juice was an effective protection against many poisons.

Ancient Greeks used it to preserve food, as a disinfectant, a water-cleansing agent, and for treating various other ailments.

The Romans used it for keeping moths out of woollen clothings, and later in cooking, and in preparation of refreshing drinks.

Properties of Lemon

- Ripe lemons have a light yellow and shiny skin.
- The half-ripe lemon has green spots and a matte skin.
- An over-ripe lemon is deep yellow or brownish yellow, very soft to the touch.
- The paler the yellow, the tarter the fruit.

- The lemon with a deep yellow skin is less sour than the others.
- The size of the fruit is not indicative of the juice it yields.
- Thin-peeled lemons are juicier than those with thick peels.

Extracting Juice from a Lemon

- It is easier to extract juice from a lemon that is kept at room temperature than from one that is kept in the refrigerator.
- To extract maximum juice easily, roll the lemon back and forth several times on a surface, using firm pressure.
- You can also get more juice by placing the lemon in an oven set at $40-50^0$C ($105-120^0$F) – an average-sized lemon should yield 2-3 tablespoons of juice.
- For extracting a small amount of lemon juice, prick a tiny hole and squeeze out the required quantity of juice, preserving the fruit for future use.

Lemon Rind and Oil

- Lemon peel, cut into strips, can be dried on some wax paper for two to three days for use later on.
- Similarly the grated rind can be dried, powdered and stored in jars.

- The white part, the inner layer of the fruit, has an extremely bitter taste.
- Once the rind has been grated, use the fruit immediately to prevent it from becoming mouldy.
- Always buy lemon oil in small quantities as it has a short shelf life – it should be stored in a dark and cool place.

How to Keep Lemon Fresh

- To keep lemon fresh, soak them in cold water for an hour each day – this will keep them fresh for five days.
- To preserve them for days together, bury them in a pot of moist sand or mud and store in air-tight containers.

Honey

Honey, one of nature's most splendid gifts to mankind, possesses unique nutritional and medicinal properties.

It has been proved that bacteria cannot live in the presence of honey because it is an excellent source of potassium which withdraws from the bacteria the formation of moisture which is essential to their very existence.

In India, honey has been used for several thousand years a an ingredient commonly found it medicines.

In Egypt too, it formed the basis of many medical preparations.

The ancient Greeks used it as a remedy for several ailments, and combined it with other foods for health-giving nourishment.

Ancient Egyptians and Greeks used honey to embalm their dead, for honey retains all its qualities even after many years.

For ages, natural honey made by the bees from nectar was the only sweetener available to man.

Though in recent years there have been many substitutes, honey still remains the dominant sweetener, offering life-rejuvenating qualities that are rarely found in any other substance.

Properties of Honey

- It is a viscous, sweet, semi-translucent liquid of golden-brown colour.
- It has an aromatic odour and a sweet taste.
- It has a tendency to become opaque and crystalline.
- Any medicine taken with honey is easily absorbed by the body system, and recovery from illness is faster, as honey has the property of acting as a catalyst to the process of absorption.
- Honey which has turned crystalline can be clear and smooth again, by standing the sealed jar in a saucepan of warm water, and gently heating to near boiling point, leaving it standing in the saucepan till it is cool.

- If honey is one of the ingredients mentioned in a recipe, warm it slightly to allow it to flow smoothly.
- A tablespoon of honey together with a small piece of ginger taken the first thing in the morning, acts as a weight-reducing agent.
- There are many countries where this wonderful gift of nature, honey, has been, and still is, used in various culinary recipes.

Nutrients Found in Lemon and Honey

Lemon

- Lemon is particularly rich in citric acid and vitamin C.
- It is mainly due to its citric acid and vitamin C contents that the lemon is widely used in medicine.
- While the pulp of a lemon contains many essential nutrients, the juice has all those nutrients in slightly less concentrated form.
- The juice yields 90 per cent of the vitamin C contained in the whole fruit.
- Two-thirds of the calcium and one-third of the iron present in the fruit is found in the juice.
- The best way to benefit from the precious nutrients is to eat the entire fruit, including the pulp.
- Two and a half lemons, including the pulp and juice, provide the average daily requirement of vitamin C and citric acid for an average adult.
- Vitamin C deficiency leads to fatigue, stress-related problems an impaired and delayed ability to heal, and a weakened immune system.

13

- Recent scientific findings reveal that an overdose of vitamin C does not lead to harmful side effects.
- Vitamin C repels free radicals and protects healthy cells from becoming cancerous, and is specially beneficial for smokers.
- Vitamin C in lemons help in converting cholesterol into primary bile acid in the small intestine.
- Lemons with their rich vitamin C content promote healing.
- Since the vitamin C in lemons stimulates the production of collagen, fractures heal better.
- Lemons promote constant regeneration and new formation of bone tissue, connective tissue and cartilage.
- Lemons stimulate the incorporation of calcium and help in the development of strong and healthy teeth.
- In lemons, bioflavonoids are mostly concentrated in the white layer between the peel and the pulp, and they carry out important biological tasks in the human organism.
- The nutrient quercetin, the most important of bioflavonoids, present in lemons, has an antibiotic and anti-allergenic effect.
- The quercetin in the lemon is a substance that prevents allergies and inflammation, as it is a sort of natural antihistamine.

- Some bioflavonoids, especially quercetin, also possess antiviral properties.
- Quercetin slows down the activity of the enzyme, aldosereductase, which stimulates the production of sorbitol, thus preventing cataract.
- The tissue of the lemon peel has 30 per cent (approximately) pectin that helps in the prevention of various heart diseases and intestinal cancers.
- The pectin in the lemon belongs to the large group of complex carbohydrates that are essential for digestion – keeps the food mash in the intestines elastic, stimulates stronger movement of intestinal muscles, and accelerates the digestive process.
- By ingesting foods rich in pectin, we follow an easy regimen to prevent being overweight, without experiencing a nagging hunger.
- Lemon increases the flavour and improves the taste of various dishes.
- It is often used in salads, as it prevents discolouration of fruits like sliced bananas and apples.
- As a natural preservative, it is often used in the preparation of cool drinks, jams, jellies, marmalades and pickles.
- Lemons also have a small amount of iron and vitamin B-complex.

Honey

- Iron, copper, manganese, silica, chlorine, calcium, potassium, sodium, phosphorus, aluminium and magnesium, all are present in honey.

- Plants absorb nutrients from the soil and use some of them to form nectar, which the bees use to form honey. Hence, the honey varies in mineral content according to the mineral resources of the soil.

- Honey contains the numerous minerals that are needed by the human body in very small amounts to maintain the mineral balance in the body.

- Dark-coloured honey is richer in copper, iron and manganese than the light-coloured ones.

- From a nutritional standpoint, iron is important because of its relation to haemoglobin.

- Copper tends to help in the absorption of iron and therefore helps in restoring the haemoglobin content of the blood in anaemic patients.

- Honey contains large amounts of pollen that are rich in vitamin C. Many vegetables lose their vitamin content while cooking, and fruits lose theirs to a marked degree during storage.

- Honey is low in thiamine, but is fairly rich in riboflavin and nicotinic acid.

- Whereas cane sugar and starches must undergo a process of inversion in the gastrointestinal tract by the action of enzymes to convert them into simple sugars, this has already been done for honey by the bees, by means of the secretion from their salivary glands, which converts the sugar in the nectar into simple sugars, levulose and dextrose, making it unnecessary for the human gastrointestinal tract to do this work.

- Honey is a predigested sugar that helps a person with a weak digestion or one who lacks the two enzymes, invertase and amylase, which help in the process of inversion.

- Besides being a welcome variation and delicious adjunct to the menu, honey is packed with the nutrients that the body needs to rejuvenate itself.

- For babies who are not breastfed, honey furnishes minerals which supplement those found in milk, as well as a small amount of protein.

- Honey is taken into the body quickly because of its dextrose content, while the levulose, being somewhat more slowly absorbed, is able to maintain the blood sugar level.

- Honey has the advantage over sugars which contain high levels of dextrose, since it prevents the raising of the blood pressure level in the body, which can be very harmful for a healthy system.

- Honey, with its high caloric content, can build up energy with smaller servings.

- Honey also contains most of vitamin B complex components – pantothenic acid, riboflavin, nicotinic acid, thiamine, pyre-doxin, biotin and folic acid.
- The sugars present in honey are glucose, fructose and sucrose.
- The glucose in honey restores the oxygen that is replaced by lactic acid when fatigue sets in.
- The fructose, also known as levulose, in honey helps the body in building up tissues.
- Dextrine is a gummy substance present in honey. The presence of dextrine in honey makes it easy to digest.

Benefits of Lemon and Honey

Lemon

- Research scientists in Argentina have discovered that lemon is a natural disinfectant for drinking water.
- Lemon oil is an excellent natural insect repellant.
- Quercetin, found in lemon, stimulates the production of insulin, which is compromised in cases of diabetes mellitus.
- The pectin in lemon supports the function of the pancreas, while stimulating the production of bile as well.
- Pectin also has the property to attract environmental toxins and digestive remnants, viruses and bacteria, and hold on to them until the digestive process is over and they are excreted.
- Pectin has the power to guard against intestinal cancer.
- Lemon acid stimulates the production of hydrochloric acid which is necessary for digestion.

- Lemon helps to stimulate the body's immune system and to prevent illness in the most natural way possible.
- The vitamin C in lemons counteracts weaknesses in the body's defences, aided in this function by bioflavonoids.
- The bioflavonoids in lemons help to maintain a high level of vitamin C in individual body cells.
- Lemons contain several nutrients that protect against various ailments.
- They can be used both internally and externally. They can be used in the form of tea, juice, masks or poultices, for they are a natural healing agents.
- A lemonade is a refreshing drink and a delicious way of quenching one's thirst.
- Dried and powdered lemon peels make an excellent tooth powder.
- Lemon oil, though bitter, has a high medicinal value as a flavouring agent and is known for its curative properties.
- It acts as a carminative that relieves flatulence.
- Lemon juice is valuable as an antiscorbutic and refrigerant.
- Lemon juice destroys the toxins in the body due to its high potassium content.
- Lemon destroys the germs responsible for diphtheria, typhoid and other deadly diseases.

- They promote bile secretion.
- The bark of the lemon tree is an antipyretic agent.
- The seeds of lemon help in expelling worms from the intestine.
- The vitamin C in lemon increases the body's resistance to various diseases.
- They promote the rapid healing of wounds.
- The presence of vitamin C in lemon prevents damage to the eyes.
- It is helpful in maintaining healthy teeth and bones as vitamin C helps in calcium absorption. It prevents decay of teeth, bleeding of gums, dental caries, and loosening of teeth.
- Lemon juice and grated rind add flavour to stewed dried fruits.
- Lemon juice serves as a substitute for vinegar.

Honey

- Honey is easily and rapidly assimilated by the body.
- It is non-irritating to the lining of the digestive tract.
- It is delicious and gives energy instantly. Hence, it is a wonderful breakfast accompaniment to start the day with.
- It enables sportspersons, who expend energy heavily, to recuperate rapidly from exertion.

- Of all sugars, honey causes the least amount of stress.
- Honey has a natural relaxative effect.
- It has a sedative quality required to calm a nervous body.
- It is easily obtainable and is inexpensive.
- It can be preserved for years without getting spoilt.
- It possesses an antiseptic and a mild laxative action.
- It has a fine flavour which increases palatability.
- It provides an infant with the composite of minerals needed for its growing body.
- Folk medicine regards honey as the best remedy of all for sleeplessness – you will observe the next morning that you must have fallen asleep very soon after your head touched the pillow.
- Ginger and honey, when taken as a cure for coughing, do not cause stomach problems as many cough syrups do.
- The intake of honey with meals is beneficial before a workout, after a workout, and during the rest-period 'jack-up' while doing the activity.
- It can be used in the daily diet without fear of having any ill-effects.
- It can be used as a natural sweetener and spread.
- It can be used in combination with such foods as fruit salad, yogurt, custards, tea, puddings, cakes, etc.

- More honey can be tolerated by the average athlete than any other of the energy foods and beverages.
- Honey is considered versatile as it can be used in many ways, and in combination with various foods and beverages.
- It is a pure food, apparently free from bacteria and other irritating substances.
- When athletes are on a weight-reducing diet, a teaspoonful of honey at the end of a meal gives a feeling of fullness, making dieting less difficult, and helping them to sustain the feeling of vigour.
- Intake of honey also prevents weight loss due to hard work and continued activity.
- Honey is one of the finest sources of producing warmth in the body.
- A mixture of honey and alcohol is believed to promote growth of hair, when it is massaged on to the scalp and allowed to remain there for two hours before rinsing off thoroughly with a mild shampoo.
- Honey acts as a natural tonic for blood.
- It is also known to provide the body with strength and vigour.

Curative Powers of Lemon

- Adding lemon juice to meals and generally using as many lemons as possible in food preparation prevents cholera infection.
- Lemon stimulates the salivary glands. Saliva helps in digestion and hence elderly people who produce inadequate amounts of saliva should take lemon.
- Lemon oil is useful for physical as well as emotional ailments.
- Lemon oil promotes spiritual well-being when used in aroma-therapy.
- In topical applications it destroys bacteria and fungi.
- Staphylococci that cause pimples, abscesses, urinary tract infection, infectious arthritis, or heart muscle infections, are destroyed within five minutes of exposure to lemon oil.
- Lemon oil also destroys *salmonella typhi,* the bacteria responsible for causing typhoid fever, approximately one hour after being treated with the oil.

- Two to three hours of exposure to lemon oil kills pneumococci that cause lung infections, meningitis, inner ear infections and peritonitis.
- The vitamin C in lemons prevents scurvy.
- It helps the body's immune system fight off viruses and bacteria by promoting the production of the protein interferon which protects cells from the harmful germs.
- Women who consume lemon regularly over a prolonged period of time have less chances of osteoporosis setting in.
- Lemon is helpful in treating stomach and digestive disorders as it is rich in vitamin C.
- Vitamin C in lemon neutralises free radicals and hence reduces the risk of cataracts by about 80 per cent.
- The average life expectancy of a person can be raised by six years by regular intake of vitamin C rich lemon and its juice.
- Eating a fresh lemon half an hour before a physical workout prevents muscle injuries and soreness after intensive exercise.
- Regular consumption of lemons along with their white inner skin reduces symptoms of allergy and slows down the production of histamine, an excessive discharge of tissue hormone, in the body.

- The bioflavonoid quercetin can be highly beneficial in preventing the formation of cataracts as a result of diabetes.
- Quercetin present in lemons protects the beta cells of the pancreas – that produce insulin against damage from the free radicals.
- The pectin in lemon, when consumed regularly, protects against cardiovascular disease by keeping the harmful LDL (low-density lipoprotein) cholesterol at low levels – this cholesterol is mainly responsible for deposits forming in blood vessels, thus thickening them, leading to heart attacks or strokes.
- Lemon acid, interacting with other acids and enzymes, ensures healthy and easy digestion.
- Lemon oil is beneficial in improving one's appetite.
- Lemons have curative properties and are hence useful for treating the following ailments:

Acne

- Boil one litre water to sterilise it.
- Cool, and stir in 2 tablespoons of honey in it.
- Add the freshly squeezed out juice of 1 lemon to it.
- Store and wash the acne-affected area with this water twice daily.

Asthma

- Take 1 tablespoon of lemon juice before meals to get relief from symptoms of asthma.

Biliousness

- Mix the juice of half a lemon in a cup of boiled and cooled water.
- Add 1 teaspoon of powdered cumin seeds.
- Powder 4 to 5 cardamoms and add to the lemon water.
- Take this concoction once every two hours to stop biliousness.

Belching

- Consume the undiluted juice of one medium-sized lemon twice a day. You can take it every day till you find relief.

Bronchitis

- Boil and then cool water to a temperature where it is still steaming but is comfortable to inhale.
- Add 1 teaspoon salt and 5 drops of lemon oil.
- Inhale thrice a day, and you will gradually find relief.
- If you experience a slight burning sensation in the throat, then mix together 100 ml freshly squeezed lemon juice and 100 ml olive oil, and take 1 teaspoon every hour.

Burning Soles and Heels

- Rub a sliced lemon all over the burning soles and heels of the feet.
- This application promotes toxin elimination through the pores of the feet.

Burning Sensation while Urinating

- Mix the juice of half a lemon in a cup of boiling water.
- Add 1 tablespoon of honey to it.
- Drink 3 cups of this water in a day to alleviate the burning sensation.

Cankers (Mouth Sores)

- In a glass of lukewarm water, mix the juice of a freshly squeezed lemon.
- Rinse your mouth frequently with this solution, or at least thrice a day.

Catarrh

- Slowly roast a ripe unpeeled lemon till it begins to crack open.
- Squeeze out 1 teaspoon juice from this lemon.
- Add ½ teaspoon honey to it.
- Take once every hour till you find relief.

Constipation

- Squeeze the juice of a lemon in a glass of warm water.

- Take this the first thing in the morning.
- You may also add 1 teaspoon honey to it as it has mild laxative properties.

Cellulite
- Mix a few drops of lemon oil with 1 tablespoon jojoba oil.
- Massage into the affected areas twice a day.

Common Cold
- Squeeze the juice of 1 lemon into a glass of lukewarm water.
- Drink a glass of this every two hours.
- Add honey if it is too sour.
- For a clogged nose, add 1 tablespoon of freshly squeezed lemon juice and a pinch of salt to a glass of lukewarm water.
- Close one nostril with a finger.
- Hold the glass of water up to the other nostril and inhale the liquid.
- Hold it for a while, then blow it out.
- Repeat with the other nostril till you find relief.
- Another form of relief is to mix the juice of two lemons in half a litre of boiling water.
- Sweeten it with 1 tablespoon honey.
- Drink a glass of this in the morning and at bedtime.

- The juice of 1 lemon, 4 teaspoons honey and ¼ teaspoon salt in a cup of warm water should be taken every night till you find relief.

Cough

- Place 2 lemons in a pot filled with water so that they are fully submerged.
- Place over a low flame for 10 minutes, taking care that the water does not boil.
- Remove the lemons and squeeze out the juice.
- Add 3 teaspoons glycerine and 250 gms honey.
- Blend well, and take 1 teaspoon of this mixture before bedtime.
- You may also take another teaspoonful of this syrup if a coughing fit should occur in the middle of the night.

Corns

- Place a thick slice of lemon on the corn, bandage and fasten.
- Repeat this application until the corn disappears.
- You may also massage 1 to 2 drops of lemon oil daily, only over the affected area.

Cystitis

- Squeeze out the juice of a lemon in a glass of boiling water.

- Cool this water.
- Drink ¼ cup of this every two hours, and it will give relief from the burning sensation as well as stop the bleeding in the cystitis.

Diarrhoea
- Boil a glass of water and cool it.
- Add the juice of a freshly squeezed lemon.
- Taking this 3 to 5 times a day will destroy the disease producing agent pathogen, thus giving relief from diarrhoea.
- To prevent the onset of diarrhoea, 1 to 2 teaspoons lemon juice should be taken before every meal.

Digestive Disorders
- Mix a teaspoon of lemon juice with 1 glass of water.
- Add a pinch of soda bicarbonate.
- This reduces acidity in the stomach and acts as a powerful carminative in case of indigestion.
- A teaspoonful of fresh lemon juice with an equal quantity of honey stops excessive accumulation of saliva in the mouth.

Dysentery
- Mix 3 teaspoons of honey with the juice of 1 lemon in a glass of water.

- This should be taken twice or thrice if the dysentery is mild.
- If it is severe, use salt instead of honey.

Ear-related Problems

- Boil equal quantities of lemon juice, sesame oil and basil juice, and let it cool a little.
- While it is still lukewarm, apply 4-6 drops of this juice in the ear twice a day for 2 days to stop the earache.
- Warm 1 teaspoon of lemon juice with 2 teaspoons of water.
- Apply a few drops in the ear to clear the ear-block.
- Apply a few drops of lemon juice in the ear to stop any discharge from the ear.

Eczema

- Add 8 drops of lemon oil with 1 tablespoon of honey.
- Add this to 1 cup of lukewarm water.
- Soak a linen cloth in this liquid and gently squeeze out the excess liquid.
- Place the cloth on the affected areas for 20 minutes.
- Repeat this treatment twice or thrice a day – this will prevent skin infection while also providing relief from the itching sensation.

- Make a paste of basil leaves to get 2-3 tablespoons of it.
- Add the juice of 2 lemons and a pinch of salt to it.
- Apply this on the affected areas.

Eye Disorders
- In the case of conjunctivitis, a few drops of warm lemon juice diluted with half a cup of water and instilled in the eyes gives relief.
- Mix together 1 teaspoon of fresh lemon juice with 4 teaspoons of rosewater.
- Washing the eyes with this water regularly, prevents old-age cataract.

Fevers
- Mix 8 drops of lemon oil with 1 tablespoon of cream and 2 cups of cold water.
- Soak a linen cloth in it and then gently squeeze out the excess liquid.
- Wrap the cloth around both calves.
- Now add several layers, using a large towel or 2 small towels.
- You can remove the wrap after 2 minutes.
- Do this at least 3 times a day, applying the cloth to both calves, till the fever has abated.
- Drinking lemon juice also brings down the fever.

Foot Relaxation

- For tired and sore feet, add a teaspoon of rock salt in hot water and soak the feet in it for 15 minutes.
- Then thoroughly rub the feet with slices of lemon.
- The contrasting action of hot water which opens the pores, and the lemon juice which has a cooling and astringent action, revitalises the feet.

Gingivitis

- Mix the fresh juice of a lemon in a glass of lukewarm water.
- Rinse the mouth thoroughly with it for at least 1 minute, so that the acid in the juice helps to dissolve the plaque and firm up the gums.

Gout

- Mix the juice of a fresh lemon in a glass of lukewarm water.
- Drink this water after each meal, as the lemon juice stimulates the formation of calcium carbonate in the body, and also neutralises the acids in the body.

Gum Disorders

- Drink a glass of diluted fresh lemon juice to which a pinch of rock salt has been added, twice a day, to relieve swollen gums.

- The rind of the lemon from which the juice has been extracted should be rubbed over the gums.
- Mix equal quantities of soda bicarbonate and salt. Add a pinch of this to a teaspoon of fresh lemon juice. Massage the gums with this juice to stop the bleeding.
- Mix ½ teaspoon of sandalpaste in a cup of warm water. Add the juice of half a lemon. Rinse the mouth with this to strengthen the weak gums and to rid the mouth of bad odour.

Hair Loss
- Cut a lemon into two and massage the scalp, ensuring that you use both the juice and rind while massaging.
- After half an hour, rinse the hair with cold water.
- Frequent massage with lemon helps in the prevention of hair loss.

Halitosis
- Squeeze the juice of 1 lemon in a glass of water.
- Thoroughly rinse your mouth several times a day, which helps to freshen breath affected by specific spices, alcohol or cigarettes.
- Chew on a slice of lemon after every meal.

Hangover
- Mix together the juice of 4 lemons, 3 tablespoons lemon-vinegar, a pinch of salt and 2 cups of lukewarm water.

- Drink on an empty stomach before breakfast, and this will help to stimulate the functioning of your stomach.
- To get relief from headache after a hangover, add the juice of 1 lemon to a cup of strong black coffee.
- Drink it unsweetened.

Hay Fever

- Scrape away the lemon peel, leaving as much white part of the lemon as possible.
- Two weeks before the usual onset of your hay fever, start eating 2 lemons peeled in this manner each day.
- If you start getting symptoms of hay fever, increase the quantity of lemon intake.
- By adding 1 to 2 tablespoons of honey with lemon, it would be more effective in preventing the onset of the hay fever.

Headache

- Mix the fresh juice of a lemon with a cup of strong black coffee.
- Drink it without milk or sweetener.
- If the pain continues, you can drink 3 cups of lemon coffee daily.
- Peel 1 large organically grown lemon.
- Squeeze the peeled rind softly between your fingers.

- Rub this moistened peel against your temples to massage the essential oil into your skin.
- Discard the layer of white skin underneath the peel.
- Press the inside of the lemon peel against your temples, and the headache should soon disappear.
- Mix equal quantities of honey and lemon juice, and drink it to cure the headache.
- For migraines, mix 100 ml jojoba oil with 20 drops lemon oil, 10 drops each of lavender oil, peppermint oil and 6 drops rosemary oil.
- Massage your temple and the nape of your neck with this oil.

Herpes
- Soak the end of a cotton bud in a drop of undiluted lemon oil, and dab the blister with it, being careful not to break open the blisters.

Hypertension
- To 1 litre milk, add 3 crushed garlic cloves and 1 chopped onion.
- Slowly bring the milk to a boil and allow it to stand for 5 minutes.
- Pour it through a strainer and cool.
- Squeeze out the juice of 3 lemons and add to the milk.
- Sip throughout the day at regular intervals.

- Cut 30 lemons into halves.
- Coat each with a thick layer of salt and dry them all in the sun.
- Powder the dried lemons.
- Take 1 teaspoon of this powder on an empty stomach every day.

Indigestion

- Mix together 1 teaspoon lemon juice and a pinch of soda bicarbonate in a glass of water.
- Drink this twice or thrice a day.

Insect Bites

- Mix together 1-2 drops of lemon oil and 1 teaspoon honey.
- Apply this tonic on the skin around the bite to prevent infection.
- Add a dash of lemon vinegar to a glass of water.
- Soak a handkerchief in this mixture and apply over the affected area.
- Add 20 drops of lemon oil to a cup of water and use it as an insect-repellent spray.
- Burn candles scented with lemon oil in your room to keep away the mosquitoes.
- If you are sitting outside, add 10 drops lemon oil to 50 ml sunflower oil, and rub all over the skin.

Jaundice

- Mash a ripe banana. Add 1 teaspoon lemon juice and 1 teaspoon honey to it, and eat it.

Joint Pains

- Mix equal quantities of lemon juice and castor oil.
- Apply this on the painful joints and massage lightly.
- Drink a glass of warm water to which 1 teaspoon each of lemon juice and honey have been added.

Lack of Concentration

- In a water-filled aromatherapy lamp, add 4 drops lemon oil.
- Breathing this air helps in alleviating lack of concentration, and is also helpful in cases of fatigue and mild depression, as the oil stimulates brain activity.
- With an atomiser, spray the room with 2 cups of water to which 15 drops of lemon oil have been added.

Liver Disorders

- Add the fresh juice of 1 lemon to a glass of warm water.
- Drink three glasses of lemon juice in a day to stimulate the liver and rejuvenate bile secretion.

Malaria

- Extract the juice from an onion.
- Mix with an equal quantity of lemon juice.
- Taking this thrice a day should bring relief from the disease.

Menstrual Disorder

- Take 1 tablespoon of lemon juice without diluting it, three or four times a day to bring excessive menstrual bleeding under control.

Nosebleed

- Squeeze out some juice from a fresh lemon. Soak a Q-tip or cotton bud in it and gently dab the inside of your nose, tilting your head slightly forward to prevent the blood from flowing into the throat – the injured blood vessels contract as soon as they come into contact with the lemon juice.

Obesity

- Mix the juice of 1 lemon with a glass of water. Add a spoon of honey and mix well. Drink this twice a day, especially in summers.

Oedema

- Mix 1 teaspoon lemon juice with a cup of tender coconut water. Drink this twice a day.

Osteoporosis

- Squeeze out the juice of 1 lemon and mix it with a glass of warm water. Add 1 tablespoon of lemon vinegar to this. Sweeten it with one tablespoon honey.
- Drink a glass of this mixture once before breakfast and again before dinner.
- Lemon juice helps in calcium absorption.

Peptic Ulcers

- Mix the fresh juice of 1 lemon with 1 glass of water.
- Drinking this twice a day helps in digestion and absorption of fats, and also in neutralising excessive bile produced by the liver as the citric acid in the lemon has an alkaline reaction in the system.

Piles

- Cut a lemon into two and coat one half with rock salt.
- Tuck this into a corner of your mouth, taking in the juice slowly.
- The lemon juice will, with its anti-haemorrhagic properties, and the magnesium sulphate-rich rock salt, check bleeding piles, help good bowel movement and gradually shrink the pile masses.
- Another cure is to mix 1 teaspoon each of lemon juice and honey with a ripe mashed banana, and eat it twice a day.

Pimples

- Boil a cup of milk. Add the juice of a lemon. Mix 1 teaspoon of glycerine in it and leave it for half an hour. Apply this on the pimples at night before going to bed.
- Gently rub a lemon peel on the pimples during daytime for 15 minutes before washing it off.
- Make a paste of the shoots of the lemon plant. Mix it with a little turmeric.
- Apply this paste on the pimples and let it stand for twenty minutes before rinsing your face.

Pregnancy-related Problems

- Drinking a cup of lemon sherbet (1 glass water, 1 teaspoon lemon juice, 6 teaspoon sugar or 2 teaspoon honey) every day will ensure easy delivery.
- Using lemon in your food daily will ensure healthy growth of the bones of the unborn baby, and protect its brain and nerve cells.

Pyorrhoea

- Squeeze out the juice of a lemon in a glass of water.
- Drink a glass of this after each meal.

Rheumatism

- Mix several drops of lemon oil with a tablespoon of jojoba oil.

- Massage the affected area with this oil to alleviate inflammation or cramps and ease the pain.
- Mix the juice of 1 lemon with a glass of lukewarm water.
- Drink this juice thrice a day.
- When the pain is acute, use the juice of 2 lemons instead of 1.

Scabies

- Mix the juice of a lemon with half teaspoon sulphur powder.
- Apply this paste on the affected area after a bath, and once before going to bed.

Scorpion Bite

- Place a crystal of potassium permanganate on the part bitten by the scorpion. Squeeze out a few drops of lemon juice over the crystal.

Scurvy

- Add the juice of 1 lemon to 3 teaspoons of water. Add half a teaspoon of honey to it.
- Drink this thrice a day – the presence of vitamin C, an appreciable quantity of vitamin B, and the healing qualities of honey make it anti-scorbutic and an excellent medicine to cure scurvy.

Enlargement of the Spleen

- Cut 2 lemons into halves.

- Coat each piece with rock salt on the cut end.
- Slightly heat each half.
- Eat these pieces during the course of the day.

Sprains

- Make a fine paste of lemon-grass.
- Mix 6 tablespoons of sesame oil with the paste.
- Boil the mixture.
- Apply this oil on the painful joints and muscles, and lightly massage for 5 minutes.

Stomachache

- Add the juice of a lemon to a glass of lukewarm water.
- Drink a glass of this with each meal, as the lemon acid stimulates the production of the enzymes in the stomach, and activates the stomach muscles.
- Powder together 1 teaspoon each of salt, dry ginger, cumin seeds and sugar.
- Mix this in half a cup of warm water.
- Add the juice of half a lemon.
- Drinking this immediately brings a lot of relief from the acute pain.

Sunburn

- Add the juice of 3 lemons to 2 cups of cold water.
- Carefully wash the areas affected by sunburn as this will cool the skin, disinfect and heal it.

- Make a poultice of 250 gms low-fat curd, 2 tablespoons clear honey and 1 tablespoon lemon juice.
- After rinsing the affected area with the lemon water (mentioned above), rub the poultice on the affected areas.
- Rinse with clear water after 15 minutes.

Tonsillitis
- Add the juice of 1 lemon to a glass of warm water.
- Gargle every 2 hours with this lemon water.
- The gargled water can be swallowed, allowing the vitamin C and bioflavonoids in the lemon juice to strengthen the immune system from within.

Toothache
- Powder 3 cloves with 1 teaspoon lemon juice.
- Apply this on the painful gums and tooth, and massage lightly.

Ulcers
- Cut a lemon into two.
- Rub the ulcerated area with the lemon in a gentle manner so as not to lacerate the skin. This can be done four to five times a day, for lime has healing properties.

Varicose Veins

- Mix together 6 drops lemon oil, 50 ml wheatgerm oil, 2 drops each of cypress and juniper oil.
- Massage the legs gently from bottom to top, always in the direction towards the heart.
- Mix 5 drops lemon oil and 1 tablespoon cream with 1 cup of warm water.
- Soak cloths in it and wrap the affected areas, leaving them on for 15 minutes.
- Keep your legs elevated during this time.
- This should be done daily as a routine.
- A lemon oil bath also helps in stimulating the blood vessels and fighting varicose veins when the legs are heavy and tired.
- Mix 6 drops lemon oil with 2 drops each of cypress oil, rosemary oil and juniper oil, and 1 tablespoon honey.
- Add this mixture to a small tub of warm water.
- Soak your legs till the knees in it for 20 minutes.

Vomiting

- Mix together 1 teaspoon of lemon juice and 1 teaspoon of sugar.
- Lick this little by little till the queasy sensation disappears.
- You can also add honey instead of sugar.

Curative Powers of Honey

- Honey has sedative properties to calm down nervous, high-strung individuals.
- It promotes sound sleep at night while calming down stressed nerves.
- It is soothing to the stomach.
- Honey provides relief from cough.
- It also provides relief from pain in arthritis because of the presence of potassium in honey.
- Honey will, by several effects, render old age less difficult to live.
- Mothers unable to nurse their babies can feed them honey which, apart from a fine flavour, has all the composite minerals needed for the baby's growing body.
- One or two teaspoonfuls used in 8 ounces of feeding mixture ensures rare chances of infants having colic.
- If the infant is having constipations, increase the amount of honey by another half teaspoon.

- If looseness of the bowels develops, the amount should be decreased by half a teaspoon.
- Giving a child a teaspoonful of honey at bedtime will help the honey to act as a sedative to the nervous system.
- If you are troubled by a cough, make use of the following cough remedy:

  Boil 1 lemon slowly for 10 minutes to soften it so that more juice can be extracted from it. Cut the lemon into two and extract the juice. Add 2 tablespoons of glycerine. Stir well, then fill up the glass bottle with the honey adding the lemon and glycerine, and stir well. A teaspoon of this can be taken whenever the need be.
- At times we may be troubled by an annoying twitching of the eyelids or at the corner of the mouth. This will soon disappear by taking 2 teaspoons of honey at the time of each meal.
- Cramps in the body muscles, occurring mostly in the legs and feet during the night, can generally be controlled by taking 2 teaspoons of honey at each meal.
- When honey is applied on burns, it relieves the painful smarting, and prevents formation of blisters.
- Honey helps the body in recovering from exertion. So athletes regain vigour faster if they take honey after a workout or exercise.

- Honey is good for students because of its rejuvenating power.
- Honeycomb is excellent for treating certain disturbances of the respiratory tract. The waxy substance in the honeycomb from which all the honey has been abstracted is used for treating certain problems of the respiratory tract.
- In folk medicine, honey is used as an anti-allergen.
- Individuals who have honeycomb until their mid-teens seldom have a cold, hay fever, or other nose disorders.
- Chewing honeycomb helps in building immunity against respiratory tract infections.
- A stuffy nose can be cured by chewing honeycomb for a few days.
- In case of a sinus attack, take one bite of honeycomb every hour for four to six hours, chewing each bite for fifteen minutes and discarding the remains of the honeycomb. The nasal passage will open up and the pain will subside.
- If honeycomb is chewed once a day for one month before the expected hay fever date, the hay fever will either not appear or will be mild in character.
- In case of a mild hay fever, the medication mentioned above taken once a day, thrice a week, will keep the nasal passage open and dry. If honeycomb is not available, take two teaspoons of honey at the time of each meal.

- In case of a moderately severe hay fever, chew honeycomb five times a day for the first two days, and thrice a day thereafter for as long as needed.
- Honey taken with milk increases the body's natural immunity against diseases.
- Honey is excellent for patients suffering from tuberculosis or diabetes.
- Apply a thick coat of honey over the mouth ulcers to cure them.
- Pain and swelling in the gums due to accumulation of pus can be alleviated by applying honey.
- Apply a mixture of honey and lemon on the swollen joints to get relief. Sprains too can be treated in a similar manner.
- A tablespoon of honey taken every night before going to bed stops excess and frequent urination.
- Babies should be given eight drops of honey and one teaspoon juice of basil leaves thrice a day, to bring cold and fever under control.
- A tablespoon of old honey, taken every day over a period of time, helps in reducing weight.
- If you feel sluggish, take a teaspoon of honey for immediate relief.

Heart Diseases
- Taking honey regularly at meal times helps patients who have arteriosclerosis or weak heart.

- Taking a glass of water with honey and lemon juice in it before going to bed is especially beneficial for heart patients.

Anaemia

- Honey with its rich source of iron, copper and manganese assists remarkably in building up the haemoglobin count in the body.
- Honey is beneficial in curing anaemia as it helps maintain the right balance of haemoglobin in the red blood corpuscles.

Eye Disorders

- Honey is an excellent cure for various eye ailments.
- Washing the eyes daily with diluted honey improves one's eyesight.
- It is beneficial in the treatment of conjunctivitis, trachoma, itching of the eyes, watery eyes, etc.
- Drinking water with honey in it, and external application of honey prevents glaucoma in the initial stage of the disease.

Insomnia

- Honey calms down high-strung nerves, and thus helps one in getting sound sleep.
- Two teaspoonfuls of honey in a cup of water, before going to bed, helps one in getting sound sleep.

- Honey can safely be given to babies for good sleep.

Irritating Cough

- Honey has a soothing effect on the inflamed mucous membrane of the respiratory tract when taken regularly.
- Honey also relieves irritating cough and difficulty in swallowing.

Old Age

- In old age, regular consumption of honey provides energy and warmths to the body.
- It helps in clearing the phlegm and mucous from the respiratory tract and rejuvenates the body.

Oral Diseases

- Applying honey over teeth and gums helps in cleaning them thoroughly.
- Mouth rinsers with honey prevents deposit of tarter at the base of the teeth, and prevents tooth decay, as honey has antiseptic qualities.
- In the case of ulcers in the oral cavity, honey helps in their early healing preventing further sepsis and pyogenic infection associated with pus formation and bad odour.
- Gargling with honey and water is beneficial in gingivitis.

Pulmonary Disorders

- Mixing honey in hot water and inhaling the steam is beneficial and soothing for asthma patients.
- Honey mixed with milk or water taken twice a day also brings relief to asthma patients.

Sexual Debility

- Honey is curative as a spermastogenic and sexual stimulant.
- It is known to strengthen the virility in men and the fertility of women.
- One part honey and three parts water mixed together and boiled together till the quantity is reduced by one-third, taken every day promotes a feeling of rejuvenation.

Stomach Disorders

- Regular intake of honey mixed with water tones up the stomach muscles, and helps in digestion.
- It also helps in decreasing and balancing the over-production of hydrochloric acid, thereby preventing nausea, heartburn and vomitting.
- Honey also acts as a laxative, and hence is beneficial for people suffering from constipation.

Storage of Lemon and Honey

Lemon

- Lemon can be stored in the refrigerator or freezer for as long as a year.
- A lemon that has been cut can be kept fresh for days if the cut end is coated with vinegar.
- When you refrigerate the lemons, ensure that there is enough space for air to circulate around the fruit on all sides – it is best to store them in wire bowls or perforated containers.
- Lemon juice can be frozen in ice-cube trays – when thawed they taste as if they were freshly squeezed.
- Lemon slices or wedges can be frozen in vacuum-sealed plastic freezer bags.
- When the whole fruit is frozen, only the juice can be used later on.
- While using lemons for cooking or storing, use only enamelled or stainless steel pots – avoid using pots made of aluminium.

Honey

- Honey should never be stored in the refrigerator or cellar as this will cause it to lose its ability to absorb, condense and retain moisture.
- It should be stored in a dry and not too warm place.
- A tightly closed container is best suited for storing honey.
- Honey can be stored in bottles, jars, vessels with lids, or tight-lid containers.
- Since honey can be stored for several years, an ideal place would be one which need not be easily accessible – keep small quantities in a reachable place for daily use.

Beauty Care

- Lemon contains many anabolic agents and nutrients that make it popular as a home remedy and useful in the preparation of natural beauty products.
- Honey has many curative properties which bring a glow to one's skin.

Skin Care

- Lemon oils and creams slow down the aging process by firming up, cleansing and regenerating the skin.
- For oily skin, blend 50 ml jojoba oil with 6 drops lemon oil and 4 drops cypress oil. Gently massage your face with this mixture every morning and night.
- Mix 1 cup jojoba oil with 1 cup olive oil. Add the peel of 2 lemons as well as their juice. Cut 4 stems of fresh lemon grass into tiny pieces and extract their juice by crushing them. Add the crushed pieces and 2 tablespoons dried lemon grass to the above mixture. Store it in a bottle of brown glass. Place the bottle in a water bath

for half an hour with the bottle open, and water at temperature of 40-50°C (105-120°F). Remove and close the lid tightly. Store for a month, shaking the bottle every second day. Strain after a month, and add 30 drops evening primrose oil. This oil is used for revitalising the skin.

- Honey, an antiseptic, hastens healing of cracks and sores, while simultaneously promoting the activity of the oil glands.

Masks and Packs

- Lemon mask is ideal for minimising wrinkles. Blend together 1 egg yolk and 15 ml jojoba oil. Add the juice of 1 lemon and rub the mixture on the wrinkles. Leave it on for 20 minutes and wash off with cold water.

- For oily skin, heat 2 cups water, and add 5 drops of lemon oil that has been mixed with 1 tablespoon cream and 1 teaspoon honey. Soak a linen in this and apply to the skin, leaving it on for 15 minutes before rinsing the face.

- For tired skin, add 5 drops lemon oil and 1 teaspoon honey to 50 gms low-fat curd, then add 2 tablespoons warm water. Mix well and apply to skin, leaving it on for 20 minutes. Gently wash and pat dry the skin.

- For dry skin, mash a ripe banana and mix with 3 drops lemon oil, 2 tablespoons each of olive oil and jojoba oil and 2 egg yolks to make a smooth paste. Apply on the skin and leave it on for 20 minutes. Rinse it with 1 litre water to which the juice of 2 lemons has been added.

Cleansing

- Mix the juice of 1 lemon with 100 ml milk and 15 ml honey. Soak a cotton ball in this mixture and gently dab the skin with it. Rinse your face after 5 minutes with plenty of warm water.

- For pimples and blackheads, blend the juice of 1 lemon with 15 ml cognac. Dip a cotton end in the solution and dab it onto the pimple affected area and blackheads several times a day.

- For rough and coarse skin, mix 1 tablespoon honey in 250 ml water. Add the juice of 1 lemon and mix well. Soak a cotton ball in the solution and apply on the rough areas of the skin of the face, hands and elbows.

Hair Care

- Lemon has some invaluable ingredients that promote a healthy scalp and hair growth.

- For greasy hair, add 5 teaspoons soapnut powder to two cups of boiling water. Cool the water to body temperature. Add the juice of 1 lemon, 2 egg yolks and 5 drops lemon oil to the water. Wash your hair with this shampoo to regulate the oil level of the scalp, and to give your hair a pleasant lemony scent.

- For long and dull hair, add the juice of a lemon to 2 cups of water, and then add 30 ml olive oil. Heat this to body temperature and massage into the scalp and hair. Wrap a towel on the head, leaving the conditioner on for 40 minutes. Then rinse thoroughly with clean water.

- Rinse your hair with the juice of half a lemon added to 1 cup lukewarm water for shiny and voluminous hair.

Baths

- Lemon juice and lemon oil added to your hot water bath refreshens and regenerates your skin, leaving it tingling and glowing.

- For skin conditioning, blend together the juice of 5 lemons, 8 drops lemon oil and 2 litres whey. Pour into your bathtub in which the temperature of water is 35°C (95°F). Soak in this water for half an hour, relishing the aroma and feel the gentle essences on your skin.

- Cut a lemon into half and place it in a bowl of water. In the morning pour this water and lemon slices in the bathtub. Add to the water 15 ml honey, 5 drops lemon oil, and 2 drops each of rosemary and eucalyptus oil. Soak in this bath for 15 minutes till you feel totally refreshed.

- For tired feet, blend together 5 drops lemon oil, 5 drops lavender oil and 1 tablespoon cream. Add all these ingredients to a bathtub of water. Soak your feet in it for 15 minutes. Massage the juice of 1 lemon into your feet after bath.

Refreshing Drinks

Spicy Lemonade

Ingredients
1 tbsp honey
3 tbsp orange juice
5 gm cinnamon
2 cloves
Rind of ½ lemon
½ l water

Method
Boil the water, cinnamon, cloves and lemon rind for nearly 2 minutes over a low heat. Combine the honey and orange juice and add to the boiled water. Mix and pour into warmed glasses. Serve immediately.

Banana Cream

Ingredients
Juice of 1 lemon
Grated rind of 1 lemon
1 cup honey
Juice of 2 oranges
3 cups water
3 bananas
2 stiffly beaten egg whites

Method
Mash and beat the bananas till creamy. Add the lemon and orange juice along with the lemon rind. Bring the water to the boil. Dissolve the honey in it. Pour it over the fruits. Mix well, and cool. Fold in the egg whites, mix and chill.

Fruit Punch

Ingredients
1 cup orange juice
2 cups grape juice
1 cup lemon juice
2 cups water
1 cup honey

Method
Combine all the ingredients together. Serve cool or chilled.

Fortifying Drink

Ingredients
1 glass water
4 cloves
4 peppercorns
1 tsp aniseed
Juice of ½ lemon
½ lemon with rind
1 tbsp honey

Method
Bring the water to the boil. Add the juice of lemon. When cool, add the honey, aniseed, peppercorns, cloves and lemon rind. Let the ingredients stand in the water for a while, then strain and serve chilled.

Egg Cocktail

Ingredients
1 egg white, beaten
1 tbsp honey
Juice of 1 orange
Juice of 1 lemon

Method
Mix together the juice of lemon and orange. Add the honey in a mixing bowl. Add the whites. Serve in cups covered with crushed ice-cubes.

Spiced Tea

Ingredients
6 cups water
2 tsp tea leaves
2 tbsp lemon juice
½ cup honey
1" piece cinnamon
A pinch of ground cloves

Method
Put all the spices in water. Warm over a low heat for 10 minutes, but do not boil. Pour it over the tea leaves slowly. Cover and steep for a minute. Filter the tea. Add the lemon juice and honey. Serve warm.

Honeyed Vodka

Ingredients
1 peg vodka
2 ice cubes
1 tsp honey
Soda water
Juice of ½ lemon

Method
Dissolve the honey in a little water in a tall glass. Add 2 ice cubes and the lemon juice. Fill with the soda water and vodka. Mix well.

Honeyed Rum

Ingredients

1 cup rum

2 tsp honey

A Pinch of cinnamon powder

Juice of 1 lemon

2 cloves

Method

Combine all the ingredients in a tall glass. Mix well and serve chilled. It can even be served as a warm drink.

Orange Lemonade

Ingredients

50 gm honey

400 ml soda water

6 tbsp orange juice

2 tbsp carrot juice

1 egg yolk

Juice of ½ lemon

2 ice cubes

Method

Mix together the honey and the egg yolk. Add the orange juice, lemon juice and carrot juice. Mix with the soda water and add the ice cubes. Serve.

Lemon Fizz

Ingredients

½ cup lemon juice
½ cup honey
2 eggs
½ cup water
½ cup ice cubes
A handful of mint leaves

Method

Mix together the lemon juice, honey, eggs, water and ice cubes in a blender. Blend till the ice crushes finely. Pour into glasses and garnish with the mint leaves.

Pineapple Cocktail

Ingredients

1 cup pineapple juice
½ cup lemon juice
2 tbsp lime juice
1/3 cup honey
1 egg white
6 ice cubes

Method

Put all the ingredients, except the ice cubes, in a blender. Blend at a high speed. Add the ice cubes and again blend till the cubes are crushed and the liquid is light and frothy. Serve chilled.

Papaya Passion

Ingredients

1 medium-sized ripe papaya
Juice of 3 oranges
Juice of 1 lemon
1 tbsp honey

Method

Cut the papaya into small cubes after peeling away the skin, and removing the seeds. Mix in a blender. Add the orange and lemon juice, and the honey. Blend again. Serve chilled.

Mixed Cocktail

Ingredients

300 gm tomatoes
1 cup water
2 tsp tomato sauce
2 tsp honey
1 tsp salt
½ tsp chilli powder
Juice of 4 oranges
Juice of 1 lemon

Method

Blanch the tomatoes and remove the skins. Run in a blender. Strain and cool. Add the rest of the ingredients and mix well. Serve with crushed ice cubes.

Holly Punch

Ingredients
1 cup honey
1 cup pineapple juice
1 cup orange juice
¼ cup lemon juice
½ l water

Method
Mix all the ingredients well. Add soda water if required. Serve chilled.

Minty Lemonade

Ingredients
4 tbsp lemon juice
1 cup honey
4 tsp ginger juice
1 tsp mint paste
1 cup soda water
A handful of mint leaves

Method
Mix together all the ingredients, adding soda water in the end. Serve with crushed ice and garnished with a few mint leaves.

Orange Delight

Ingredients
1 ½ cups orange juice
2 tsp grated orange rind
2 tbsp lemon juice
1 cup honey
2 egg whites
2 tsp gelatine

Method
Beat the egg whites till stiff. Dissolve the gelatine in a little water. Add all the ingredients to it and mix thoroughly. Chill and serve.

Whisky Froth

Ingredients
1 peg whisky
2 pegs lemon juice
2 tbsp honey
2 ice cubes

Method
Mix together all the ingredients in a blender. Blend on high speed for 10 seconds. Serve immediately.

Watermelon Refresher

Ingredients

6 cups watermelon cubes
¼ cup honey
1 tbsp lemon juice

Method

Mix all the ingredients in a blender, and run for a few seconds. Serve chilled.

Pomegranate Juice

Ingredients

4 cups pomegranate juice
1 cup water
2 tbsp honey
½ lemon
Ice cubes

Method

Dissolve the honey in water. Add it to the pomegranate juice. Squeeze the lemon juice into it and top it up with the ice cubes.

Honey Delight

Ingredients

1 glass chilled milk

4 almonds

4 cashew nuts

4 pistachios

1 tbsp cream

2 tbsp honey

A pinch of powdered cardamom

Method

Make a paste of the nuts. Stir into the milk. Add the honey and cardamom powder and stir well. Top it up with the cream. Serve chilled.

Lemony Lime

Ingredients

2 sweet limes

2 lemons

4 tbsp honey

5 cups cold water

Ice cubes

A pinch of black salt

A pinch of pepper powder

Method

Extract the juice of the limes and lemons. Add all the other ingredients and stir well. Serve chilled.

Mango Treat

Ingredients

2 cups mango juice
1 tbsp honey
Grated rind of ½ lemon
Juice of ½ lemon
4 ice cubes
A pinch of nutmeg powder

Method

Mix together all the ingredients. Serve chilled with the ice cubes.

Honey Fizz

Ingredients

4 tbsp honey
2 tbsp lime cordial
1 tbsp sugar syrup
Juice of ½ lemon
A few pineapple cubes

Method

Stir together all the ingredients into a tall glass. Garnish with the pineapple cubes.

Rummy Cola

Ingredients
3 tbsp rum
1 bottle cola drink
1 tsp honey
Juice of ½ lemon
1 egg white
10 gm chocolate, grated

Method
Pour the rum in a jug. Add the cola drink, honey and lemon juice and stir well. Beat the egg white till stiff and blend into the drink. Pour in two glasses. Top each glass with the chocolate and serve chilled.

Lime-Wine Melody

Ingredients
90 ml white wine
30 ml lime cordial
100 ml chilled soda
1 tsp honey
Juice of ½ lemon
8 seedless green grapes
2 ice cubes

Method
Mix together all the ingredients, except the grapes and pour into tall glasses. Add the ice cubes and top it up with the grapes.

Fruity Buttermilk

Ingredients

2 cups buttermilk

1 tsp orange juice

1 tbsp pineapple juice

1 tbsp honey

Juice of ½ lemon

250 ml soda water

10 ice cubes

Method

Blend together all the ingredients and serve immediately.

Milk Cocktail

Ingredients

1 tbsp honey

½ cup milk

4 tbsp carrot juice

Juice of ½ lemon

1 tbsp orange juice

2 tbsp crushed ice

Method

Mix together all the ingredients in a blender. Run the blender for 30 seconds. Serve immediately.

Apple Cocktail

Ingredients

3 apples

50 gm honey

200 ml milk

3 tsp pineapple juice

1 lemon wedge

2 ice cubes

Method

Mix all the ingredients, except the lemon wedge, and blend for 30 seconds. Garnish with the lemon wedge and serve immediately.

Rich Fruity Cocktail

Ingredients

2 cups milk

2 tbsp orange juice

1 egg yolk

1 small banana

6 almonds, slivered

4 tbsp honey

3 ice cubes

Method

Pour all the ingredients in a blender. Blend for 30 seconds. Serve immediately.

Ice Cream Cocktail

Ingredients
1 scoop chocolate ice cream
1 scoop vanilla ice cream
50 gm honey
20 gm chocolate, grated
1 glass milk

Method
Warm the milk, adding the chocolate and honey. Remove from the heat and allow it to cool. Pour into a mixing bowl. Add the ice creams. Whisk for 30 seconds. Serve immediately.

Gooseberry Juice

Ingredients
4 tbsp gooseberry juice
4 tbsp honey
Juice of 2 lemons
1 cup cold water

Method
Mix together all the ingredients. Chill before serving.

Cucumber Juice

Ingredients
Juice of 2 large cucumbers
Juice of 2 lemons
½ cup honey
1 cup buttermilk
Ice cubes
A dash of salt and pepper

Method
Mix together all the ingredients and serve chilled.

Egg Fizz

Ingredients
1 egg yolk
1 cup cold milk
2 tsp honey
1 cup soda water
½ tsp vanilla essence

Method
Whisk the egg yolk and honey into the milk until frothy. Add the vanilla essence. Pour into tall glasses and top with the soda water. Serve immediately.

Pineapple Sherbet

Ingredients

2 glasses buttermilk
4 tbsp honey
1 cup pineapple, crushed
½ tsp cardamom powder
Juice of ½ lemon
Ice cubes

Method

Mix together the buttermilk and honey till the honey dissolves. Add the pineapple and cardamom. Stir well. Then add the lemon juice and ice cubes, and run in a blender till the ice cubes are crushed. Serve immediately or refrigerate till used.

SECRET GUIDES

This series of guides lets you into the secrets of better health care and also gives you an insight into the causes of diseases and the ways to cure them.

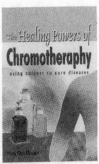

The Healing Powers of
Chromotheraphy
Hari Om Gupta
Rs. 150

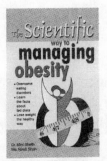

The Scientific way to
Managing Obesity
Mini Sheth & Ms. Nirali S.
Rs. 150

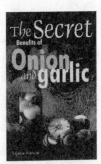

The Secret Benefits of
Onion and Garlic
Vijaya Kumar
ISBN 1 84557 533 4
Rs. 75

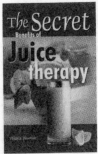

The Secret Benefits of Juice
Therapy
Vijaya Kumar
ISBN 1 84557 535 0
Rs. 75

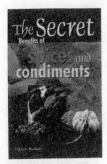

The Secret Benefits of
Spices and Condiments
Vijaya Kumar
ISBN 1 84557 585 7
Rs. 75

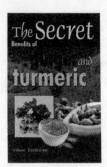

The Secret Benefits of
Ginger and Turmeric
Vikaas Budhwaar
ISBN 1 84557 593 8
Rs. 75

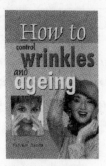

How to Control Wrinkles
and Ageing
Parvesh Handa
ISBN 1 84557 607 1
Rs. 99

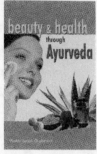

Beauty and Health through
Ayurveda
Vaidya Suresh Chaturvedi
Rs. 75

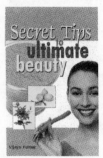

Secret Tips to Ultimate
Beauty
Vijaya Kumar
ISBN 1 84557 532 6
Rs. 75

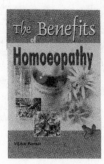

The Benefits of
Homoeopathy
Vijaya Kumar
ISBN 1 84557 626 8
Rs.75

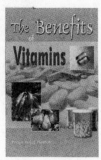

The Benefits of Vitamins
Pooja Bajaj Malhotra
ISBN 1 84557 645 4
Rs. 75

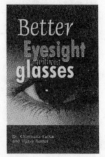

Better Eyesight without
Glasses
Dr. Chinthana Patkar
ISBN 1 84557 444 3
Rs. 75

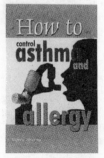

How to Control Asthma and
Allergy
Rajeev Sharma
ISBN 1 84557 534 2
Rs. 75

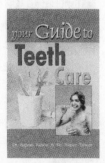

Your Guide to Teeth Care
*Dr. Rajesh Talwar &
Dr. Nupur Talwar*
ISBN 1 84557 591 1
Rs. 75